MICHELLE LISTIAK

ANXIETY RELIEF NOW

Easy & Effective Techniques to Feel Better Fast

Contents

Introduction

In today's fast-paced world, anxiety has become an all-too-common experience for many of us. Whether it arises from the pressures of work, the uncertainty of the future, past events or the demands of daily life, anxiety can feel overwhelming, leaving us trapped in a cycle of worry and fear. It's important to recognize that anxiety is not a sign of weakness, but rather a natural response to stress. However, when left unchecked, it can interfere with our well-being, relationships, and overall quality of life.

The good news is that anxiety can be managed. This book is designed to provide you with a toolbox of practical, effective techniques to help you navigate and reduce anxiety in your life. From simple breathing exercises to more in-depth mindfulness practices, each chapter offers strategies backed by science and time-tested wisdom. Whether you're looking for quick relief in moments of panic or long-term strategies to help prevent anxiety from taking hold, you'll find something here to suit your needs.

The journey to feeling calmer, more centered, and in control begins with small, consistent steps. As you explore the techniques outlined in this book, remember that there's no "one-size-fits-all" approach. What works best for you may require some experimentation, but with patience and practice, you'll be able to regain balance and build resilience against life's stresses.

Together, let's take the first step toward understanding your anxiety, discovering the relief you deserve, and living a more peaceful, fulfilling life.

1

Techniques to Use Anytime Anywhere

DOUBLE EXHALE BREATHING

The **Double Exhale Breathing Technique** is a simple yet powerful method that focuses on lengthening the exhale to twice the duration of the inhale. This practice promotes relaxation, reduces stress, and improves the balance between the body's nervous systems.

How To Do Double Exhale Breathing:

1. **Inhale**: Begin by inhaling through your nose for a count of 4 seconds. Focus on breathing deeply into your diaphragm, expanding your belly rather than your chest.
2. **Exhale**: Once your inhale is complete, exhale gently through your mouth or nose for a count of 8 seconds. The key here is to exhale slowly and fully, releasing tension with each breath out. (Note: if the 4-8 count feels too long, begin with inhaling for 2 seconds and exhaling for 4 seconds.)
3. **Continue**: Repeat this cycle for several minutes, gradually increasing the duration as you become more comfortable. Aim for

a steady rhythm where your exhalation is always twice as long as your inhalation.

Benefits of Double Exhale Breathing:

- **Calms the Nervous System**: The extended exhale activates the parasympathetic nervous system, which is responsible for the body's "rest and relax" response. This leads to reduced stress levels and a sense of calm.
- **Improved Oxygen Exchange**: By lengthening the exhale, the technique encourages more complete expulsion of carbon dioxide, which may enhance the efficiency of oxygen exchange in the lungs.
- **Increases Mindfulness**: This breathing method demands concentration and presence, helping you become more aware of your body and mind. It can be a valuable tool for meditation or grounding techniques.
- **Enhanced Relaxation**: The controlled, prolonged exhalation has been shown to reduce heart rate, lower blood pressure, and induce a deeper state of relaxation. This makes it an excellent technique for use before sleep or during stressful situations.

When to Use Double Exhale Breathing:

- **Before Sleep**: Practicing this technique before bedtime can help calm the mind and prepare the body for restful sleep.
- **During Stressful Situations**: Whether you're dealing with anxiety, tension, or frustration, the double exhale can quickly restore a sense of calm.
- **In Meditation**: This technique can be integrated into mindfulness or meditative practices to deepen your focus and sense of well-being.

Tips for Double Exhale Breathing:

- Maintain a comfortable, upright posture to allow your lungs to fully expand.
- If you find it difficult to inhale or exhale for the desired duration, start with shorter counts (e.g., inhale for 2 seconds, exhale for 4 seconds) and gradually work your way up.
- Practice regularly to train your body to respond to stress with deeper, slower breaths.

This technique is simple to learn and can have significant physical and mental health benefits when practiced regularly. Whether you're looking to enhance relaxation, improve focus, or reduce anxiety, the Double Exhale Breathing Technique is an excellent tool for promoting overall well-being.

DIAPHRAGMATIC BREATHING

Diaphragmatic breathing is a natural, deep-breathing technique that engages the diaphragm, a large muscle located beneath your lungs, to promote more efficient and fuller breaths. This technique emphasizes breathing from the abdomen, rather than shallow chest breathing, which is common when we are stressed or anxious. By encouraging deeper, slower breaths, diaphragmatic breathing helps activate the parasympathetic nervous system, inducing relaxation and improving overall health.

How to Do Diaphragmatic Breathing:

1. **Find a Comfortable Position**: Start by sitting or lying down in a comfortable position. Ensure your back is straight, your shoulders are relaxed, and your hands are resting on your abdomen.
2. **Inhale Slowly**: Breathe in deeply through your nose, allowing your diaphragm to expand. As you inhale, imagine your belly moving forward (if sitting) or rising up (if lying down) as air fills your lungs from the bottom up. The goal is to make the abdomen (not the chest) expand outward as you breathe in.
3. **Exhale Fully**: Slowly exhale through your mouth, allowing your belly to release inward (if sitting) or down (if lying down). This ensures that the diaphragm is fully engaged, releasing out as much air as possible. Continue the exhale until you've expelled all the air from your lungs.
4. **Repeat the Process**: Continue breathing slowly and deeply, focusing on the movement in and out (if sitting) or the rise and fall (if lying down) of your belly. Aim for a steady rhythm and relaxed pace. Gradually, you can lengthen the duration of both the inhale and the exhale as you become more comfortable with the technique.

Benefits of Diaphragmatic Breathing:

- **Reduces Stress and Anxiety**: By engaging the diaphragm and activating the parasympathetic nervous system (the "rest and digest" system), diaphragmatic breathing helps to lower the body's stress response, decreasing heart rate and blood pressure.
- **Improves Lung Capacity**: This technique encourages fuller, deeper breaths, which improves oxygen intake and promotes more efficient use of the lungs, enhancing overall lung health and capacity.

- **Promotes Relaxation**: Diaphragmatic breathing helps trigger the relaxation response in the body. It calms the mind, reduces feelings of anxiety, and improves focus, making it an excellent tool for mindfulness and meditation.
- **Improves Posture**: By focusing on engaging the diaphragm and using the muscles of the abdomen, diaphragmatic breathing promotes better posture and helps alleviate tension in the neck and shoulders, which are often associated with shallow chest breathing.
- **Helps with Sleep**: Practicing diaphragmatic breathing before bed can help reduce the physical symptoms of stress, calm the mind, and prepare the body for restful, deep sleep.
- **Enhances Digestion**: As diaphragmatic breathing stimulates the abdominal organs and reduces stress, it can also support better digestion and relieve symptoms of indigestion or bloating.

When to Use Diaphragmatic Breathing:

- **During Stressful Moments**: If you feel overwhelmed or anxious, diaphragmatic breathing can help restore calm by slowing your heart rate and promoting a sense of safety.
- **In Meditation or Mindfulness**: This technique can be an integral part of meditation practices, helping you deepen focus and presence.
- **Before Sleep**: It can be a calming pre-sleep practice to help your mind and body unwind.
- **To Improve Athletic Performance**: Athletes use diaphragmatic breathing to enhance endurance, improve oxygen flow, and promote recovery after exercise.

Tips for Effective Diaphragmatic Breathing:

- **Practice Regularly**: The more you practice diaphragmatic breathing, the more natural it will become. Try incorporating it into your daily routine.
- **Breathe from Your Belly**: Focus on the movement of your abdomen rather than your chest. If needed, place one hand on your chest and the other on your belly to ensure that your abdomen is moving primarily.
- **Be Patient**: If you're not used to breathing this way, it might feel strange at first. With time, you'll find that it becomes easier and more natural.

Common Mistakes to Avoid with Diaphragmatic Breathing:

- **Shallow Breathing**: Be mindful not to fall back into shallow chest breathing. Focus on making your abdomen move with each breath.
- **Holding Your Breath**: Some people tend to hold their breath as they focus on the technique. Aim for a smooth, continuous flow of inhalation and exhalation without pausing.
- **Tensing Your Body**: Keep your shoulders, jaw and neck relaxed. Tension in the upper body can hinder the natural flow of diaphragmatic breathing.

Diaphragmatic breathing is a simple yet powerful technique that supports physical and mental well-being. By engaging the diaphragm, it enhances lung function, reduces stress, promotes relaxation, and fosters mindfulness. Whether you're looking to manage anxiety, improve your posture, or prepare for a restful night's sleep, diaphragmatic breathing is an excellent tool to incorporate into your daily life.

JIN SHIN JYUTSU

Jin Shin Jyutsu is an ancient Japanese healing art that involves using gentle touch on specific points of the body, called safety energy locks, to promote balance and relieve physical and emotional stress. This technique is based on the idea that the body's energy flows through pathways, and by tapping into these energy flows, you can restore harmony and alleviate symptoms like anxiety.

How Jin Shin Jyutsu Helps with Anxiety:

Jin Shin Jyutsu works on the principle that energy blockages in the body can lead to emotional imbalances, such as anxiety, stress, and fear. By gently holding specific points on the hand, this technique aims to release these blockages and restore the flow of energy, resulting in a sense of calm and emotional equilibrium. Some of the most effective techniques in this practice involve working with the fingers/thumbs, which play a significant role in both physical and emotional healing. These techniques help restore harmony between the body and mind, fostering a greater sense of peace and emotional balance.

Key Techniques:

1. **Thumb Hold**: In Jin Shin Jyutsu, each finger corresponds to a particular emotion or organ system. The thumb is associated with the stomach and spleen, and it is linked to feelings of **worry, anxiety, and stress**. Holding the thumb gently can help release tension and anxiety. This action can help calm the mind and relieve anxiety by balancing the energy of the stomach and spleen.
2. **Index Finger Hold**: One of the simplest yet most effective techniques in Jin Shin Jyutsu involves working with the index finger. The index finger is associated with **fear, self-doubt**, and

also corresponds to the stomach and spleen. Working with this finger can help release tension and emotional blockages related to these areas, supporting a sense of security, clarity, and calm. The index finger is believed to influence not only the physical body (particularly the digestive system) but also the emotional state. By holding the index finger, we are said to release fear and anxiety, clear negative emotions, and improve energy flow throughout the body. In this technique, the energy blockages tied to the stomach, spleen, and emotions like fear and worry are gently released, leading to a sense of emotional balance and peace.

3. **Ring Finger Hold**: The ring finger is associated with **grief, sadness, letting go** and the lungs and large intestine. The energy flow in the ring finger is connected to the body's ability to release grief, sadness, and emotional pain. It is also believed to support the respiratory system and the elimination processes in the body. Holding the ring finger is thought to support emotional release, especially when dealing with difficult emotions such as sorrow, loss, or unexpressed grief, improve your respiratory function, and restore balance to your body's energy flow. By working with the ring finger, you can release emotional blockages, clear tension in the lungs, and promote a sense of emotional release and physical relaxation.

How to Do Jin Shin Jyutsu:

1. **Hold the Thumb/Finger.** With one hand, gently wrap your fingers completely around the thumb/finger of your other hand applying light pressure and making sure it's not forceful or uncomfortable. The touch should be gentle and soothing.

2. **Focus on Your Breath**: As you hold your thumb/finger, take slow, deep breaths. Focus on the breath flowing in and out, allowing your

body to relax with each exhale. Inhale deeply through your nose and exhale slowly through your nose/mouth. The deep breathing enhances the effectiveness of the technique by helping to release tension from the body and calm the mind.

3. **Hold for a Few Minutes**: Keep your hold for several minutes, ideally 5-10 minutes, or until you begin to feel a shift in your emotional or physical state. You can do this technique on both hands or on just one hand if preferred. You may feel a sense of relief or emotional release as you continue to hold. Allow yourself to relax and focus on the calming energy that flows through your body.

4. **Release Gently**: When you're ready to finish, slowly release the hold on the finger/thumb and take a few more deep breaths. Notice any changes in your body or emotional state — you may feel a sense of relaxation, calm, lightness or emotional relief.

Benefits of Jin Shin Jyutsu:

- **Reduces Stress and Promotes Calmness**: By facilitating the smooth flow of energy in the body, Jin Shin Jyutsu helps calm the nervous system and alleviate feelings of anxiety and tension.

- **Balances the Emotional State**: The technique helps release negative emotions like worry, fear, and stress, which are often associated with anxiety. It promotes emotional equilibrium, helping you feel more grounded and centered.

- **Supports Deep Relaxation**: As the energy blockages are cleared, the body enters a state of deep relaxation. This allows the body to rest and heal, which is essential in reducing anxiety symptoms.

- **Improves Self-Awareness**: Regular practice of Jin Shin Jyutsu encourages mindfulness and body awareness. It helps you connect with your inner self, making it easier to identify and release anxiety triggers.

- **Holistic Approach to Mental and Physical Health**: Jin Shin Jyutsu works not only on relieving the symptoms of anxiety but also addresses the root causes by restoring balance to the body's energy systems. This holistic approach supports both mental and physical well-being.

When to Use Jin Shin Jyutsu:

- **During Anxiety Attacks**: If you're experiencing heightened anxiety, you can use Jin Shin Jyutsu self-care techniques to calm your nerves and bring your body back to a balanced state.
- **Before Stressful Situations**: Practice Jin Shin Jyutsu before a stressful event or challenge to create a sense of calm and relaxation.
- **Daily Relaxation Practice**: Incorporating Jin Shin Jyutsu into your daily routine can help you manage chronic anxiety and reduce its impact on your life.
- **As Part of a Holistic Approach**: Combine Jin Shin Jyutsu with other relaxation techniques like deep breathing, meditation, or yoga to enhance its effectiveness.

Tips for Practicing Jin Shin Jyutsu:

- **Stay Consistent**: Practice regularly to see the cumulative benefits of this technique. Even just a few minutes of self-care each day can be effective in reducing anxiety over time.
- **Be Gentle with Yourself**: Jin Shin Jyutsu is about self-care and relaxation. Be gentle with your body and allow the energy to flow naturally, without force.
- **Breathe Deeply**: Pair Jin Shin Jyutsu with deep breathing exercises to enhance its calming effects. Focus on slow, deep breaths to bring

your body and mind into a state of relaxation.

- **Trust the Process**: Jin Shin Jyutsu works on an energetic level, and the results may not always be immediately noticeable. Trust the process and give yourself time to experience its benefits.

Jin Shin Jyutsu offers a powerful, holistic approach to managing anxiety. Through gentle touch on specific energy points, this technique promotes balance in the body's energy systems, helping to release tension, calm the nervous system, and restore emotional harmony. Whether you're dealing with acute anxiety or chronic stress, practicing Jin Shin Jyutsu can help create a sense of peace and well-being. By incorporating this technique into your self-care routine, you can manage anxiety more effectively and support your overall mental and emotional health.

2

Techniques to Use at Home

THREE-PART BREATHING

Three-part breathing, also known as Dirga Pranayama or Complete Breath, is a simple yet powerful breathing technique that can help alleviate anxiety by promoting relaxation and improving focus. It involves engaging the full capacity of the lungs through a deliberate and controlled filling of the lungs in three distinct phases: the belly, the ribs and the chest in that order. This technique helps to calm the nervous system, reduce stress, and center the mind.

How to Do Three-Part Breathing:

1. **Find a Comfortable Position**: Start by sitting comfortably, either cross-legged on the floor or on a chair with your feet flat on the ground. Keep your spine straight and your shoulders relaxed. You can also lie down if that feels more comfortable.

2. **Close Your Eyes and Relax**: Gently close your eyes to minimize distractions and begin to focus on your body and breath. Take a few moments to settle in.

3. **Inhale into the Belly (Lower Lungs)**: Begin by taking a slow,

deep breath in through your nose, allowing your belly to expand like a balloon. Imagine filling the lower part of your lungs first. Place both hands on your belly and feel it move forward as you inhale. This phase of the breath engages the diaphragm, which is responsible for deep breathing.

4. **Inhale into the Ribs (Mid-Lungs):** As you continue your inhale, move your hands to the sides of your ribs and expand your ribcage up and out to the sides like bucket handles lifting and gently draw in more air. Imagine filling the middle part of your lungs.

5. **Inhale into the Chest (Upper Lungs)**: Finally, move your hands to the top of your chest and continue inhaling to fill the top of your lungs, lifting your chest upward. This phase completes the deep breath, filling the lungs from the bottom to the top. Your chest and collarbones may slightly lift as you breathe in fully.

6. **Exhale Slowly and Completely**: Once you've inhaled fully, exhale slowly and completely through your mouth or nose, emptying the air from top to bottom. First, let the chest deflate, then the ribs, and finally, the belly. Make sure the exhale is slow, smooth, and steady to promote relaxation.

7. **Repeat for Several Minutes**: Continue this three-part breathing cycle for 3-5 minutes, or longer if needed. Focus on the smooth flow of the breath and the sensations of relaxation with each inhale and exhale.

Benefits of Three-Part Breathing:

- **Activates the Parasympathetic Nervous System:** Three-part breathing stimulates the parasympathetic nervous system (the "rest-and-digest" system), which is responsible for promoting relaxation and reducing the effects of stress. When practiced regularly, this breathing technique can help balance the body's stress response and counteract feelings of anxiety.

- **Calms the Mind and Body**: By focusing on the breath and engaging the full lung capacity, three-part breathing induces a state of mindfulness. This mindfulness reduces mental chatter, allowing the practitioner to shift attention away from anxious thoughts and focus on the present moment.

- **Promotes Deep Breathing and Oxygen Flow**: Anxiety often leads to shallow, rapid breathing, which can increase feelings of panic and stress. Three-part breathing encourages deep, diaphragmatic breathing, which ensures that more oxygen reaches the brain and vital organs, promoting a sense of calm and well-being.

- **Balances Energy**: The technique helps regulate energy levels, preventing feelings of being overwhelmed, fatigued, or hyper-alert, all of which are common during anxiety episodes.

- **Reduces Physical Tension**: Many people experience physical tension during times of anxiety, especially in the shoulders, chest, and abdomen. Three-part breathing helps release this tension by encouraging relaxation throughout the entire body.

- **Promotes Emotional Calmness**: By slowing down the breath and focusing on the sensations of the body, three-part breathing creates a sense of emotional stability. This practice can be particularly helpful during moments of acute anxiety or panic attacks, helping to restore a sense of control.

- **Enhances Focus and Mental Clarity**: The practice of focusing on each part of the breath can also improve concentration and mental clarity. By directing attention to the breath, three-part breathing reduces mental distractions and allows for a deeper state of mindfulness.

- **Improves Sleep Quality**: Three-part breathing can be a helpful tool for those struggling with anxiety-related sleep disturbances. The deep, slow breaths trigger a relaxation response that can make it easier to fall asleep and stay asleep.

Tips for Practicing Three-Part Breathing

- **Practice Regularly**: While three-part breathing can be effective during moments of anxiety, it can also be beneficial to practice it regularly as part of a daily relaxation routine. The more you practice, the easier it becomes to use this technique when anxiety arises.
- **Focus on the Breath**: If your mind starts to wander during practice, gently bring your attention back to the breath. Focusing on the expansion and release of your belly, ribs, and chest can help you stay grounded and calm.
- **Use it During High-Stress Moments**: In moments of high stress or anxiety, try using three-part breathing as a way to regain calm and composure. If you're experiencing a panic attack or overwhelming anxiety, use the technique to slow down your breathing and reestablish control.
- **Combine with Other Relaxation Practices**: Three-part breathing can be even more effective when combined with other anxiety-reducing practices, such as meditation, mindfulness, or yoga. Pairing breathing exercises with a peaceful environment can enhance the relaxation response.

Research has shown that controlled breathing techniques like three-part breathing can have a positive impact on anxiety and stress levels. Studies suggest that deep, slow breathing can lower cortisol (the stress hormone) levels, reduce heart rate, and activate the parasympathetic nervous system, leading to a sense of relaxation. This technique has been used in mindfulness and yoga practices for centuries to promote mental and physical well-being.

Three-part breathing is a simple, effective technique for managing anxiety by encouraging deep, diaphragmatic breathing, promoting mindfulness, and activating the body's relaxation response. By practicing this technique regularly, you can develop a powerful tool for calming the mind and reducing physical tension during moments of stress. Whether you use it during an anxiety episode or as part of a daily relaxation routine, three-part breathing can support your overall mental and emotional well-being.

BOX BREATHING TECHNIQUE

Box breathing, also known as square breathing, is a simple yet powerful breathing technique that promotes relaxation, focus, and mental clarity. It involves consciously controlling your breath in a structured pattern of equal counts, creating a "box" shape with your inhales, holds, exhales, and holds again. This technique helps regulate the nervous system, reduce stress, and improve concentration, making it particularly useful in high-pressure situations or moments of anxiety.

How To Do Box Breathing:

1. **Inhale (4 counts)**: Begin by inhaling deeply through your nose for a count of 4. As you breathe in, expand your abdomen and allow your lungs to fill completely. Focus on a slow, steady inhale without rushing the breath.
2. **Hold (4 counts)**: After inhaling, hold your breath for a count of 4. This pause allows your body to absorb the oxygen and helps you become more mindful of the breath in your body.
3. **Exhale (4 counts)**: Slowly exhale through your mouth for a count of 4. Ensure that the exhale is controlled and steady, fully releasing the air from your lungs.

4. **Hold Again (4 counts)**: After exhaling, hold your breath again for a count of 4. This brief pause completes the "box" and prepares you for the next round of breathing.

5. **Repeat**: Continue this cycle for several minutes, focusing on maintaining a steady rhythm of equal counts for each part of the breath (inhale, hold, exhale, hold). You can adjust the count if necessary (e.g., 3 counts or 5 counts), but the key is to maintain equal durations for each phase.

Benefits of Box Breathing:

- **Reduces Stress and Anxiety**: By regulating the breath and slowing down the breathing rate, box breathing activates the parasympathetic nervous system, promoting a state of calm and reducing feelings of stress and anxiety.

- **Improves Focus and Concentration**: Box breathing helps to sharpen mental clarity by providing a rhythmic structure to the breath. This can be particularly helpful for improving concentration during work, study, or meditation.

- **Balances the Nervous System**: The even pattern of box breathing helps balance the sympathetic ("fight or flight") and parasympathetic ("rest and digest") nervous systems, reducing the body's physical stress response and promoting relaxation.

- **Enhances Mental Clarity and Performance**: Many athletes, performers, and individuals in high-pressure roles use box breathing to calm their nerves and improve mental performance, especially before important events or presentations.

- **Improves Respiratory Function**: Box breathing encourages full, deep breaths that engage the diaphragm and promote more efficient oxygen exchange, supporting lung health and overall respiratory function.

When to Use Box Breathing:

- **During Stressful Situations**: Whether you're preparing for a big presentation, dealing with a challenging situation, or experiencing anxiety, box breathing helps restore calm and clarity.
- **Before or After Meditation**: Box breathing can be used as a grounding practice before meditation or as a way to transition out of meditation to clear your mind.
- **In High-Pressure Moments**: If you're facing a stressful task, public speaking, or any situation where you need focus and calmness, box breathing can help center you.
- **To Improve Sleep**: Using box breathing before bed can help calm the nervous system and prepare the body for restful sleep.

Tips for Effective Box Breathing:

- **Maintain a Relaxed Posture**: Sit or lie in a comfortable position with your spine straight and your shoulders relaxed. This allows for optimal lung expansion during inhalation.
- **Breathe Gently**: Avoid forcing the breath. The goal is to breathe comfortably, with control and mindfulness, not to overexert yourself.
- **Focus on the Rhythm**: Try to maintain a steady, smooth rhythm in your breaths. If 4 counts feel too long or too short, adjust to a count that feels natural, but always ensure the inhale, hold, exhale, and hold are equal in duration.
- **Practice Regularly**: The more you practice box breathing, the more effective it will become in helping you manage stress, improve focus, and cultivate relaxation.

Common Mistakes to Avoid:

- **Holding Your Breath Too Long**: Avoid holding your breath for too long, as it could lead to discomfort. Stick with the recommended count (such as 4 seconds) and focus on relaxation.
- **Shallow Breathing**: Ensure that you are taking full, deep breaths, using your diaphragm. Shallow chest breathing will reduce the benefits of the technique.
- **Rushing Through It**: Try to maintain a calm and measured pace with your breaths. The goal is to slow down, not to hurry through the process.

Box breathing is a simple but highly effective technique that helps promote calm, clarity, and mental focus. By following the equal-length pattern of inhale, hold, exhale, and hold, you can reduce stress, balance your nervous system, and improve both mental and physical performance. Whether you're seeking relaxation, focus, or stress relief, box breathing is an excellent tool to incorporate into your daily life or practice in moments of need.

ALTERNATE NOSTRIL BREATHING (NADI SHODHANA)

Nadi Shodhana (also known as Alternate Nostril Breathing) is a powerful yogic breathing technique that can be incredibly effective for alleviating anxiety. The practice involves alternately breathing through one nostril at a time while closing off the other nostril, creating a sense of balance and calm within the body and mind. Nadi Shodhana works by regulating the breath, calming the nervous system, and promoting a state of mindfulness. Nadi Shodhana can be practiced anywhere, and it is especially effective when done in a quiet space where you can focus.

How to Do Alternate Nostril Breathing/Nadi Shodhana:

1. **Find a Comfortable Position:** Sit in a comfortable, upright position, either cross-legged on the floor or on a chair with your feet flat on the ground. Keep your spine straight and shoulders relaxed. You can also sit in a meditative posture or lie down if you prefer.

2. **Close Your Eyes:** Gently close your eyes to eliminate distractions and bring your attention inward.

3. **Prepare Your Hand:** Use your right hand to close your nostrils. You will use your thumb to close your right nostril, and your ring finger to close your left nostril. Your index and middle fingers can rest gently on your forehead or between your eyebrows.

4. **Begin with a Deep Exhale:** Start by exhaling completely through both nostrils.

5. **Inhale through the Left Nostril:** Close your right nostril with your right thumb and inhale deeply and slowly through the left nostril, filling your lungs completely. Focus on making the inhale smooth and even.

6. **Close the Left Nostril and Exhale through the Right Nostril:** Once you've fully inhaled through the left nostril, close the left nostril with your ring finger and release the right nostril. Exhale fully and slowly through the right nostril.

7. **Inhale through the Right Nostril:** Now, inhale slowly and deeply through the right nostril, filling your lungs completely.

8. **Close the Right Nostril and Exhale through the Left Nostril:** Close the right nostril with your right thumb, release the left nostril, and exhale completely through the left nostril.

9. **Repeat the Cycle:** This completes one cycle of Nadi Shodhana. Continue this alternating nostril breathing for 5–10 minutes, maintaining a smooth, slow, and steady rhythm with each inhale

and exhale.

10. **End with a Full Exhale:** To finish, exhale completely through the left nostril and sit quietly for a moment, observing the effects of the practice.

Benefits of Alternate Nostril Breathing/ Nadi Shodhana

- **Balances the Nervous System:** Nadi Shodhana is known for its ability to balance the sympathetic (fight-or-flight) and parasympathetic (rest-and-digest) nervous systems. By alternating the breath between the nostrils, this technique creates a sense of harmony in the body, which helps reduce stress and anxiety.

- **Calms the Mind:** Anxiety often causes the mind to race with worries and overwhelming thoughts. Nadi Shodhana brings focus to the breath, redirecting attention away from anxious thoughts and promoting a peaceful, focused state of mind. The rhythmic and controlled breathing encourages the body and mind to enter a relaxed state, reducing mental agitation.

- **Increases Oxygen Flow and Detoxifies the Body:** The practice of alternate nostril breathing enhances the flow of oxygen to the brain and vital organs, helping to clear any blockages in the body's energy channels (or "nadis," which are pathways of prana or life force). This cleansing process can help reduce feelings of tension and anxiety.

- **Regulates the Breath:** Anxiety often causes shallow, rapid breathing (also called "chest breathing"). Nadi Shodhana encourages slow, deep, and controlled breaths, which activates the parasympathetic nervous system, lowering heart rate and reducing physical symptoms of anxiety, such as rapid breathing and elevated blood pressure.

- **Reduces Stress:** By regulating the breath, Nadi Shodhana helps to activate the body's natural relaxation response, reducing the physical symptoms of stress, such as a racing heart and shallow breathing.

- **Enhances Mental Clarity:** The practice of focusing on the breath and coordinating nostril breathing can help quiet the mind, improving mental clarity and focus. This can be especially beneficial during moments of anxiety when scattered thoughts make it hard to concentrate.
- **Balances Energy:** Nadi Shodhana is said to balance the flow of energy (prana) through the body's energy channels, helping to clear any blockages and bring a sense of equilibrium. This balance helps create a feeling of calm and stability, both physically and emotionally.
- **Improves Sleep:** By calming the nervous system and reducing anxiety, Nadi Shodhana can also improve sleep quality. The practice induces relaxation, making it easier to fall asleep and stay asleep, especially if practiced before bedtime.

When to Use Alternate Nostril Breathing

- **To Reduce Stress and Anxiety:** Practice during moments of high stress or tension to promote calm and mental clarity.
- **Before Meditation or Yoga:** Use it as a preparatory technique to center the mind and enhance focus.
- **To Improve Sleep:** Incorporate it into your bedtime routine to relax and prepare the body for rest.
- **To Enhance Concentration:** Practice before tasks requiring mental sharpness, such as studying or creative work.
- **During Emotional Overwhelm:** Use it to regain balance during moments of emotional intensity.
- **To Boost Energy:** Practice in the morning or during an afternoon

slump to energize and refresh the mind.

- **To Support Respiratory Health:** Use it to strengthen and balance the respiratory system during moments of congestion or shallow breathing.
- **After Physical Activity:** Practice to cool down and regulate the breath after a workout.
- **As a Daily Wellness Routine:** Incorporate it into your daily schedule to maintain overall balance and mental clarity.

Tips for Practicing Nadi Shodhana

- **Practice Regularly:** For the best results, make Nadi Shodhana a regular part of your routine. Practicing daily, even for just a few minutes, can help reduce chronic anxiety and promote long-term mental well-being.
- **Use Nadi Shodhana During Anxiety Attacks:** If you're experiencing an anxiety attack or heightened stress, Nadi Shodhana can be a powerful tool to calm the body and mind. It can be done anywhere, even in stressful situations, to bring your focus back to the breath and reduce anxiety.
- **Start Slowly:** If you're new to the practice, start with shorter sessions and gradually work your way up to longer ones. Aim for about 5 minutes of practice, and increase the duration as you become more comfortable with the technique.
- **Focus on Slow, Deep Breaths:** Make sure each breath is slow and deliberate. Avoid rushing through the practice, and focus on maintaining a calm, steady rhythm with each inhale and exhale.
- **Combine with Meditation or Mindfulness:** Nadi Shodhana can be combined with meditation or mindfulness practices for even deeper relaxation. Pair it with a mantra or focus on the sensations of the breath to enhance the calming effects.

Research has shown that deep breathing exercises like Nadi Shodhana can significantly reduce stress, anxiety, and even lower blood pressure. Studies suggest that alternate nostril breathing may help reduce cortisol (the stress hormone) levels and stimulate the parasympathetic nervous system, which is responsible for relaxation. Nadi Shodhana is also linked to improved focus, better emotional regulation, and enhanced overall well-being.

Nadi Shodhana is an effective and accessible technique for managing anxiety. By engaging in this simple practice of alternating nostril breathing, you can balance your nervous system, calm your mind, and reduce the physical symptoms of anxiety. Regular practice can lead to long-term benefits, such as improved emotional stability, enhanced mental clarity, and a greater sense of inner peace. Whether you use it as a daily practice or during moments of heightened stress, Nadi Shodhana can be a valuable tool in your anxiety-relief toolkit.

3

Techniques for Sleep

Breathwork techniques and practices, particularly those introduced in Chapters 1 and 2, are not only effective tools for managing anxiety and stress but also have significant benefits for improving sleep quality. The practices of deep breathing, mindfulness, and specific breathing exercises help to calm the nervous system, regulate emotions, and reduce physical tension, all of which are key factors in achieving restful, restorative sleep. Below is an exploration of how some of the breath techniques covered in these chapters also promote better sleep:

Double Exhale Breathing (Chapter 1)

Double exhale breathing is a highly effective technique for enhancing sleep quality. Its benefits stem from its ability to promote relaxation and create optimal conditions for restorative rest. Here are the three primary reasons this method supports better sleep:

- **Activates the Parasympathetic Nervous System:** The extended exhalation signals the body to shift from a state of alertness (sympathetic dominance) to a state of relaxation (parasympathetic dominance). This shift helps reduce heart rate, lower blood pressure, and prepare the body for sleep.

- **Reduces Stress and Anxiety:** By focusing on a slow, controlled breathing rhythm, double exhale breathing reduces the production of stress hormones like cortisol. This helps calm racing thoughts and physical tension, common barriers to falling asleep and staying asleep.

- **Enhances Oxygen Exchange and Brain Calmness:** The longer exhale improves carbon dioxide release and enhances oxygen delivery to the brain. This supports a sense of mental clarity and calmness, essential for transitioning into deep, restorative sleep cycles.

Practicing double exhale breathing before bed creates a soothing ritual that naturally prepares the mind and body for rest, making it a powerful tool for improving sleep hygiene.

Diaphragmatic Breathing Technique (Chapter 1)

Deep breathing exercises are essential for reducing anxiety and promoting relaxation, which is key to falling asleep and staying asleep. Techniques such as diaphragmatic breathing, where you engage your diaphragm for slower and deeper breaths, activate the parasympathetic nervous system—the body's "rest and digest" system. This shift away from the "fight or flight" response helps to:

- **Calm the Mind:** By slowing down your breath and focusing on the sensation of the inhale and exhale, deep breathing can quiet the mind. This helps to create a mental environment conducive to sleep by reducing the clutter of racing thoughts that often keep people awake at night.

- **Relax the Body:** Deep breathing releases physical tension in the muscles and reduces stress hormone levels, which can often disrupt sleep. When you engage in slow, deep breathing before bed, it prepares your body to unwind and enter a state of relaxation, helping to ease into sleep more easily.
- **Regulate Heart Rate:** Deep breathing lowers your heart rate, which is crucial for falling asleep. The slower pace of breathing signals to your body that it is time to rest, contributing to a smooth transition from wakefulness to sleep.

Three-Part Breathing (Chapter 2)

Three-part breathing involves breathing deeply into three distinct sections of the body: the belly, ribs, and chest. This technique promotes relaxation by encouraging full, deep breaths, which are beneficial for sleep:

- **Promotes Deep Relaxation:** By consciously breathing into each section of the body, you activate the diaphragm and deepen the breath, which encourages the parasympathetic nervous system to engage. This lowers stress and tension, making it easier to fall asleep.
- **Calms the Mind:** The rhythmic nature of three-part breathing helps to center your focus and quiet the mind. This helps you let go of any anxious or intrusive thoughts that may interfere with sleep, making it easier to drift off.
- **Reduces Physical Tension:** As you focus on deep breathing, your body naturally begins to release tension in the muscles, which can help ease any discomfort or restlessness that might prevent sleep.

Box Breathing (Chapter 2)

Box breathing is a structured technique where you inhale for a count of four, hold for four, exhale for four, and hold again for four before repeating the cycle. This method has numerous benefits for sleep:

- **Promotes Relaxation:** The structured rhythm of box breathing helps slow the heart rate and quiet the mind. This steady pattern of breathing can be a form of mindfulness, allowing you to let go of any thoughts that may be causing restlessness or anxiety, which can often interfere with sleep.
- **Reduces Stress:** By balancing the breath and promoting deep, steady inhalations and exhalations, box breathing can lower cortisol levels, the stress hormone that is often elevated during stressful or anxious moments. Lower stress levels can make it easier to wind down and fall asleep.
- **Triggers the Relaxation Response:** Box breathing can trigger the body's relaxation response, signaling that it is time for sleep. This can make it easier to fall asleep faster and enjoy a more restful night's sleep.

Alternate Nostril Breathing/Nadi Shodhana (Chapter 2)

Nadi Shodhana, or alternate nostril breathing, is a practice that balances the energy in the body and calms the nervous system. It involves alternating the breath between each nostril while using your fingers to block one side of the nose at a time. This technique is highly effective for promoting sleep:

- **Balances the Nervous System:** By calming both sides of the brain and balancing the autonomic nervous system, alternate nostril breathing encourages a sense of peace and harmony within the body. This balance is essential for transitioning into sleep and can help quiet the mind before bedtime.

- **Reduces Anxiety:** As a gentle and focused breathing exercise, Nadi Shodhana reduces feelings of anxiety, which can often keep individuals awake at night. By slowing down the breath and clearing the mind, this practice can reduce the mental chatter that interferes with sleep.
- **Promotes Relaxation:** The slow, deep breaths and the focus on alternating nostrils help activate the parasympathetic nervous system, which promotes a state of relaxation and calm. This relaxation is crucial for preparing the body to fall asleep.

How These Breath Techniques Contribute to Better Sleep

All the breath techniques discussed in Chapters 1 and 2 help by addressing the physiological and psychological aspects that contribute to anxiety and poor sleep: These techniques and practices are incredibly beneficial for improving sleep quality. By calming the nervous system, reducing anxiety, and promoting relaxation, these breathing exercises help create the ideal conditions for falling asleep and staying asleep. Whether it's through double exhale breathing, box breathing, alternate nostril breathing, or other practices, incorporating these techniques into your bedtime routine can lead to more restful, restorative sleep and improve overall well-being.

JOURNALING OR FREE WRITING BEFORE SLEEP

Journaling or free writing before bed is a powerful and effective practice for relieving anxiety and promoting better sleep. Writing provides a safe and structured way to express emotions, process thoughts, and clear the mind, helping to reduce the mental clutter that often prevents restful sleep. When used consistently, journaling can become a valuable tool to manage stress and anxiety, leading to improved emotional well-being and a more peaceful night's rest.

How to Use Journaling or Free Writing Before Sleep:

1. **Create a Calm Environment:** To get the most out of your journaling practice, it's important to create a quiet, relaxing environment. Dim the lights, eliminate distractions, and set aside time for yourself to reflect without interruptions. This creates a peaceful atmosphere that can help ease anxiety and promote relaxation.

2. **Start with a Short Time Frame:** If you're new to journaling, start with just 5 to 10 minutes of writing. The goal is to create a regular practice, not to pressure yourself into writing for an extended period of time. Even a brief session can help clear your mind and reduce anxiety before bed.

3. **Write Freely Without Judgment:** The beauty of free writing is that it's unstructured and spontaneous. Allow yourself to write whatever comes to mind, without worrying about grammar, spelling, or punctuation. This is not about writing perfectly—it's about expressing your thoughts and emotions honestly and openly. Don't censor yourself; let the words flow freely, as this can be incredibly cathartic and relieve emotional tension.

4. **Write About Your Day:** A simple way to start journaling is to write about your day. Reflect on what happened, how you felt, and what you experienced. Identify moments of joy or satisfaction as well as any challenges or stress. Acknowledging both the positive and negative aspects of your day can help you process your emotions, reducing anxiety and improving your ability to

relax before sleep.

5. **Explore Your Worries:** If anxiety is preventing you from sleeping, try writing about your worries. Write them down in as much detail as needed, and explore what's causing the anxiety. Sometimes, just putting these thoughts on paper can help you see them more objectively, reducing their power over you. Afterward, you can ask yourself questions like: "Is this worry valid? What can I do about it tomorrow? Can I release this for now?" This helps to prevent overthinking and encourages a mindset of calm.

6. **Write Gratitude or Positive Affirmations:** Journaling doesn't always have to be about expressing anxiety. You can also focus on gratitude or write positive affirmations before bed. Reflect on things you're grateful for or repeat calming affirmations such as "I am at peace" or "I am safe and supported." Writing down these positive thoughts shifts your focus away from anxiety and fosters a sense of calm and relaxation, making it easier to drift off to sleep.

7. **Use Prompts to Guide Your Writing:** If you don't know where to start, journaling prompts can help guide your thoughts. Here are a few prompts you can use: What is weighing on my mind right now? What is something that brought me peace today? What am I grateful for today? What do I need to release before going to sleep?

8. **End with a Positive Note:** As you wrap up your journaling session, end on a positive or soothing note. This could be a sentence of self-compassion, a hopeful affirmation, or a reminder that it's okay to let go of the day's stress. Ending on a positive thought can help transition your mind into a state of relaxation, setting the stage for better sleep.

Benefits of Journaling Before Sleep:

- **Improved Sleep Quality:** By offloading anxious thoughts onto paper, journaling helps prevent those thoughts from lingering and disrupting sleep. When you release your worries through writing, you create space for relaxation, making it easier to fall asleep and stay asleep.

- **Enhanced Emotional Regulation:** Journaling helps you process your emotions and recognize patterns in your thinking. By understanding the root of your anxiety, you can learn to manage your emotions more effectively, reducing the likelihood of nighttime anxiety.

- **Increased Self-Awareness:** Writing regularly fosters a deeper connection with your inner world. Over time, journaling helps you become more aware of your triggers, thoughts, and emotional responses. This self-awareness enables you to approach anxiety with greater insight and control.

- **Relief from Overthinking:** When anxiety leads to overthinking, it's difficult to quiet the mind. Journaling helps stop the cycle of overthinking by providing a structured outlet for your thoughts. Once the thoughts are on paper, they no longer have to swirl around in your mind, allowing your brain to rest and prepare for sleep.

How Journaling Helps Relieve Anxiety

- **Clears the Mind:** One of the main causes of anxiety at night is the racing thoughts that keep people awake. These thoughts can stem from unresolved worries, tasks left unfinished, or concerns about the future. Journaling allows you to express these thoughts on paper, helping to "empty" the mind of worries. Writing down your thoughts provides an outlet for what may be troubling you, giving you a sense of relief and helping to quiet the mental noise that often prevents sleep.

- **Encourages Emotional Release:** Anxiety often involves suppressed emotions, such as fear, frustration, or sadness. Writing allows you to explore these emotions in a safe, non-judgmental space. By expressing your feelings through journaling, you release pent-up emotions, which helps to lighten your emotional load and reduce anxiety. This emotional release can bring a sense of relief, allowing you to enter a more relaxed state before bedtime.

- **Identifies and Challenges Negative Thoughts:** Anxiety is often fueled by irrational or exaggerated thoughts. Journaling provides the opportunity to identify these thoughts and reflect on their validity. By writing them down, you can begin to challenge their accuracy and replace them with more balanced perspectives. This process of cognitive restructuring can be incredibly powerful, as it helps reduce the intensity of anxious thoughts and encourages a more rational, calming mindset before sleep.

- **Provides Perspective:** Writing about your day, both its challenges and successes, can offer a new perspective on your situation. It helps to put things into context and reminds you of what went well, even in the midst of stress or anxiety. This shift in perspective allows you to see the bigger picture and prevents the cycle of negative thinking that often accompanies anxiety. By acknowledging both your struggles and triumphs, journaling provides a sense of balance and encourages a more peaceful state of mind.

- **Promotes Mindfulness:** Journaling is an inherently mindful practice. When you write, you focus on the present moment, which helps to shift your attention away from worries about the past or future. This mindfulness practice allows you to become more aware of your feelings, thoughts, and physical sensations, reducing anxiety by keeping you grounded in the present. It also encourages self-compassion, as you acknowledge your thoughts and feelings without judgment, fostering a sense of acceptance and peace.

Journaling or free writing before sleep is an effective and therapeutic tool for managing anxiety. By allowing yourself to express your thoughts and emotions without judgment, you can reduce mental clutter, challenge negative thoughts, and process emotional tension. Whether you write about your day, your worries, or your gratitude, journaling helps bring clarity and calm to the mind, making it easier to fall asleep and experience restful, restorative sleep. This simple yet powerful practice can be a valuable part of your nighttime routine, helping you to manage anxiety and promote overall emotional well-being.

How Not Eating at Least 2 to 3 Hours Before Sleep Relieves Anxiety

The timing of your meals can play a significant role in how well you sleep and how you manage anxiety. Avoiding food intake for a minimum of 2 to 3 hours before sleep is a simple yet effective practice that can help calm the mind and promote a more restful night. This practice allows your body to focus on digestion and prepares you for a deeper, more relaxing sleep by minimizing disruptions that can exacerbate anxiety.

How Eating Before Bed Can Affect Anxiety

- **Digestive Discomfort:** When you eat a large meal too close to bedtime, your body is still working to digest the food when you lie down. This can cause discomfort, such as bloating, indigestion, or acid reflux, which can make it harder to relax. The physical discomfort may trigger feelings of restlessness and irritability, intensifying anxiety and preventing the body from achieving a relaxed state. By waiting at least 2 to 3 hours after eating before going to bed, you allow your body to finish the majority of the digestive process, minimizing these disruptive sensations.

- **Blood Sugar Fluctuations:** Eating late at night, particularly meals high in sugar or carbohydrates, can lead to fluctuations in blood sugar levels, which may disrupt sleep and contribute to feelings of anxiety. As your body processes food, blood sugar levels rise and then fall, which can cause feelings of irritability, jitteriness, and fatigue—common symptoms of anxiety. By giving your body time to regulate blood sugar levels before sleep, you reduce the likelihood of these fluctuations affecting your mood and sleep quality.

- **Impact on Sleep Hormones:** The timing of meals can also influence the production of hormones that regulate sleep and stress. Eating too close to bedtime may interfere with the natural release of melatonin, the hormone responsible for helping you fall asleep. Additionally, the body's focus on digesting food can trigger the release of cortisol, the stress hormone, making it more difficult to unwind and relax. By avoiding eating at a minimum of 2 to 3 hours before sleep, you help facilitate the natural hormone balance that encourages deep, restorative sleep and minimizes anxiety.

How Not Eating Before Sleep Can Help Relieve Anxiety

- **Reduces Stress Hormones:** After eating, your body increases its production of insulin to process glucose, which can activate the sympathetic nervous system (the "fight or flight" response). This may raise levels of cortisol, which contributes to feelings of anxiety. By waiting a few hours after eating, the body's stress response is less likely to be triggered, allowing the parasympathetic nervous system (the "rest and digest" system) to take over, helping you relax more deeply.

- **Promotes Better Sleep:** When the body is focused on digesting food, it's harder to reach a state of restful sleep. Digestion requires energy and blood flow to the stomach, which can interfere with the body's natural ability to wind down and fall asleep. By waiting at least 2 to 3 hours after eating, your body can focus on relaxation and rest rather than digesting food. This promotes a deeper sleep cycle, allowing for more rejuvenating and restorative sleep, which in turn helps manage anxiety.

- **Improves Blood Sugar Stability:** Eating late at night can cause a rapid rise and subsequent drop in blood sugar, which can make you feel jittery, irritable, and anxious. By allowing your body time to stabilize blood sugar levels before sleep, you minimize the likelihood of experiencing these fluctuations. Stable blood sugar levels promote emotional stability and a calm mood, making it easier to manage anxiety both during the night and the following day.

- **Supports the Digestive System:** Digestion is a complex process that requires time and energy. Eating right before bed can lead to indigestion, heartburn, or acid reflux, as the body struggles to process food while you lie down. These physical discomforts can trigger or worsen feelings of anxiety, especially for those already prone to stress. By avoiding eating a minimum of 2 to 3 hours before bed, you allow your digestive system to work efficiently and without interference, creating a sense of physical ease and mental calmness that helps reduce anxiety.

- **Promotes Mindful Eating:** Establishing a routine where you avoid eating late at night encourages mindful eating during the day. When you give yourself enough time to digest and enjoy your meals earlier in the day, you are more likely to make healthier food choices, which can have a direct impact on your mental well-being. Well-balanced meals help stabilize your energy levels and provide the nutrients needed to manage stress effectively, thereby reducing the chances of anxiety-building triggers like sugar crashes or caffeine overload.

How to Implement This Practice

1. **Plan Your Meals and Snacks:** Try to finish your last meal or snack at least 2 to 3 hours before bed. This gives your body enough time to process the food and prepare for sleep. Plan your meals earlier in the day so you're not hungry close to bedtime. If you do need a snack later in the evening, opt for something light and easily digestible, such as a small handful of nuts.

2. **Avoid Caffeine and Sugary Foods:** Caffeine and foods high in sugar can disrupt sleep and exacerbate anxiety, especially if consumed too close to bedtime. Avoid caffeine in the afternoon and evening, and try to limit high-sugar foods at night. This will help stabilize your blood sugar levels and reduce the risk of anxiety or restlessness at night.

3. **Establish a Consistent Routine:** Creating a consistent eating and sleeping schedule can help regulate your body's internal clock. Stick to regular meal times and aim to finish eating at least 2 to 3 hours before you plan to sleep. This consistency supports better digestion and relaxation, which can help reduce anxiety and improve sleep quality over time.

4. **Listen to Your Body:** While avoiding food right before sleep can be beneficial, listen to your body's needs. If you find yourself truly hungry before bed, opt for a small, healthy snack that won't disrupt your digestive process. It's important to balance the need for relaxation with taking care of your body's nutritional requirements.

Not eating at least 2 to 3 hours before sleep is an effective way to relieve anxiety and promote relaxation. By giving your body time to digest and stabilize blood sugar levels, you reduce physical discomfort, balance hormone production, and enhance your ability to unwind before sleep. This practice not only helps reduce anxiety and stress in the moment but also contributes to better sleep quality, allowing your body and mind to fully recharge for the day ahead.

4

Food and Anxiety

Food and blood sugar levels play a significant role in influencing anxiety. The relationship between the two is complex and involves how our bodies process nutrients and how these processes impact our mental state. Here's an outline for how food and blood sugar can affect anxiety:

Blood Sugar Fluctuations and Anxiety

- **Blood Sugar Spikes and Crashes:** Rapid changes in blood sugar levels can have a direct impact on mood and anxiety. When blood sugar rises too quickly after eating sugary or carbohydrate-rich foods, it can lead to a quick energy spike. However, this is often followed by a crash, causing feelings of irritability, fatigue, and anxiety. These fluctuations can trigger the body's stress response, causing physical symptoms such as a racing heart and shallow breathing.

- **Hypoglycemia (Low Blood Sugar):** When blood sugar levels drop too low, it can lead to a condition called hypoglycemia. Symptoms of hypoglycemia include shakiness, dizziness, confusion,

41

and irritability, all of which are linked to anxiety. The body perceives hypoglycemia as a stressor, leading to an increase in adrenaline and cortisol levels, which can exacerbate feelings of anxiety.

Food Choices and Their Impact on Anxiety

- **Refined Sugars and Processed Foods:** Diets high in refined sugars and processed foods contribute to blood sugar instability. These foods can lead to spikes and crashes in blood sugar, which, as mentioned earlier, are associated with anxiety. Furthermore, processed foods often lack the essential nutrients that support brain function and emotional regulation, leading to an increased susceptibility to anxiety.
- **Complex Carbohydrates and Fiber:** Foods rich in complex carbohydrates (e.g., whole grains, vegetables, and legumes) help maintain stable blood sugar levels. Fiber slows the absorption of sugar into the bloodstream, preventing drastic fluctuations in blood sugar that could trigger anxiety. These foods also provide a steady source of energy, which can help reduce irritability and feelings of stress.
- **Healthy Fats and Proteins:** Omega-3 fatty acids found in fatty fish (like salmon and mackerel) and nuts and seeds have been shown to improve brain health and reduce inflammation, both of which are important for managing anxiety. Protein-rich foods (e.g., eggs, lean meats, legumes) can also help stabilize blood sugar and keep mood swings at bay by providing a slow and steady release of energy.

The Gut-Brain Connection

The gut microbiome, which consists of trillions of bacteria and other microorganisms, plays a crucial role in regulating mood and mental health. The food we eat can influence the diversity and composition of our gut bacteria. A balanced, nutrient-dense diet helps maintain a healthy gut microbiome, which, in turn, supports brain health and reduces anxiety.

Studies have shown that an imbalance in gut bacteria, often caused by poor diet, can lead to inflammation and affect the production of neurotransmitters like serotonin, which plays a key role in regulating mood. A lack of certain nutrients (e.g., magnesium, B vitamins) can also contribute to anxiety.

Caffeine and Alcohol

- **Caffeine:** While caffeine is commonly consumed to increase alertness, it can exacerbate anxiety in some people. Caffeine stimulates the nervous system and can cause physical symptoms like a racing heart, jitteriness, and heightened stress, all of which can contribute to or worsen anxiety.
- **Alcohol:** Although alcohol may initially seem to calm the nerves, it can disrupt blood sugar levels and sleep patterns. Over time, regular alcohol consumption can lead to blood sugar imbalances and increase anxiety symptoms. Alcohol also interferes with neurotransmitter production and disrupts the balance of serotonin and dopamine in the brain.

Nutrient Deficiencies and Anxiety

Certain nutrient deficiencies can contribute to anxiety. For example, low levels of magnesium, B vitamins (especially B12 and folate), and vitamin D have been associated with increased anxiety. Magnesium, in particular, has a calming effect on the nervous system, and its deficiency can make the body more sensitive to stress.

A balanced diet contributes to mental and emotional well-being. Eating a varied, nutrient-dense diet, rich in whole foods like fruits, vegetables, lean proteins, healthy fats, and complex carbohydrates, supports the body's ability to maintain balanced blood sugar levels and produce the neurotransmitters necessary for mood regulation.

The Importance of Regular, Balanced Meals

Skipping meals or going too long without eating can lead to blood sugar imbalances that trigger anxiety. Eating regular, balanced meals helps prevent blood sugar dips and crashes, and provides the body with a steady supply of nutrients that support brain function and mental health.

Combining protein, healthy fats, and fiber in meals can help promote sustained energy and minimize the risk of mood swings and anxiety.

In conclusion, the foods we eat and our blood sugar levels have a profound effect on our anxiety. Maintaining stable blood sugar through balanced meals, rich in complex carbohydrates, healthy fats, and proteins, can help reduce anxiety symptoms. Additionally, avoiding excessive sugar, processed foods, and alcohol, while ensuring adequate nutrient intake, supports mental well-being. By paying attention to both diet and blood sugar regulation, individuals may be able to better manage their anxiety and improve their overall mental health.

45

5

Conclusion

Effectively managing anxiety requires a holistic approach that integrates multiple strategies for mental, emotional, and physical well-being. Breathwork, such as controlled breathing techniques, helps regulate the nervous system, promoting a state of calm and reducing stress. Jin Shin Jyutsu, an ancient Japanese healing art, offers gentle, self-administered touch techniques to harmonize energy flow, fostering relaxation and emotional balance.

Journaling serves as a powerful tool for processing thoughts, identifying triggers, and cultivating gratitude, enabling individuals to gain perspective and clarity.

Additionally, maintaining a balanced diet supports emotional health by stabilizing blood sugar levels and providing essential nutrients for optimal brain function.

Together, these practices form a comprehensive toolkit for managing anxiety. By integrating these techniques into daily life, individuals can build resilience, reduce stress, and cultivate a deeper sense of inner peace.

If this book was helpful, I would greatly appreciate it if you would leave a favorable review on Amazon so others may experience the benefits of these techniques as well.

6

Resources

Aucoin, M., LaChance, L., Naidoo, U., Remy, D., Shekdar, T., Sayar, N., Cardozo, V., Rawana, T., Chan, I., & Cooley, K. (2021). Diet and Anxiety: A scoping review. Nutrients, 13(12), 4418. https://doi.org/10.3390/nu13124418

Balban, M. Y., Neri, E., Kogon, M. M., Weed, L., Nouriani, B., Jo, B., Holl, G., Zeitzer, J. M., Spiegel, D., & Huberman, A. D. (2023). Brief structured respiration practices enhance mood and reduce physiological arousal. Cell Reports Medicine, 4(1), 100895. https://doi.org/10.1016/j.xcrm.2022.100895

Banushi, B., Brendle, M., Ragnhildstveit, A., Murphy, T., Moore, C., Egberts, J., & Robison, R. (2023). Breathwork Interventions for Adults with Clinically Diagnosed Anxiety Disorders: A Scoping Review. Brain Sciences, 13(2), 256. https://doi.org/10.3390/brainsci13020256

Bentley, T. G. K., D'Andrea-Penna, G., Rakic, M., Arce, N., LaFaille, M., Berman, R., Cooley, K., & Sprimont, P. (2023). Breathing Practices for Stress and Anxiety Reduction: Conceptual Framework of Implementation Guidelines based on a systematic review of the published literature. Brain Sciences, 13(12), 1612. https://doi.org/10.3390/brainsci13121612

Chung, N., Bin, Y. S., Cistulli, P. A., & Chow, C. M. (2020). Does the proximity of meals to bedtime influence the sleep of young adults? A Cross-Sectional Survey of University students. International Journal of Environmental Research and Public Health, 17(8), 2677. https://doi.org/10.3390/ijerph17082677

Clarke, J., MD. (2016, March 23). Soothe Your Nervous System with 2-to-1 Breathing. https://yogainternational.com/article/view/soothe-your-nervous-system-with-2-to-1-breathing/?srsltid=AfmBOortPe56 0LictZCQGktSEPzxXXYc3JaW6DYGBsQ_8U3Mf7XMiKrC

Professional, C. C. M. (2024, May 1). Diaphragmatic breathing. Cleveland Clinic. https://my.clevelandclinic.org/health/articles/9445-diaphragmatic-breathing

Resources, H. (2023, June 21). Breathing for relaxation. Human Resources. https://hr.duke.edu/wellness/mental-health-stress/success-over-stress/relaxation-techniques/breathing-relaxation/

Jsjnz_Jw_Admin. (n.d.). Jin Shin Jyutsu self help. Jin Shin Jyutsu NZ. https://jsjnz.co.nz/self-help-charts/

Lamke, D., Catlin, A., & Mason-Chadd, M. (2014). Not just a theory: the relationship between Jin Shin Jyutsu® Self-Care training for nurses and stress, physical health, emotional health, and caring efficacy. Journal of Holistic Nursing, XX–XX, 1–12. https://www.jsjinc.net/ns/ups/web-articles/Julia.pdf (Original work published 2014)

Lmarchie. (2023, August 21). PART 4: EATING TOO CLOSE TO BEDTIME | TMJ & Sleep Therapy Centre of Cleveland. TMJ & Sleep Therapy Centre of Cleveland. https://clevelandtmjsleep.com/part-4-eating-too-close-to-bedtime/?utm_source=chatgpt.com

Find out how food and anxiety are linked. (n.d.). Mayo Clinic. https://www.mayoclinic.org/diseases-conditions/generalized-anxiety-disorder/expert-answers/coping-with-anxiety/faq-20057987

Ms, J. L. (2022, November 30). The 8 best breathing techniques for sleep. Healthline. https://www.healthline.com/health/breathing-exercises-for-sleep?utm_source=chatgpt.com

Nestor, J. (2020). Breath: The New Science of a Lost Art. Penguin.

Smyth, J. M., Johnson, J. A., Auer, B. J., Lehman, E., Talamo, G., & Sciamanna, C. N. (2018). Online Positive Affect Journaling in the Improvement of Mental Distress and Well-Being in General medical patients with Elevated Anxiety Symptoms: a preliminary randomized controlled trial. JMIR Mental Health, 5(4), e11290. https://doi.org/10.2196/11290

Telles, S., Vishwakarma, B., Gupta, R. K., & Balkrishna, A. (2019). Changes in shape and size discrimination and state anxiety after Alternate-Nostril Yoga breathing and breath awareness in one session each. Medical Science Monitor Basic Research/Medical Science Monitor. Basic Research, 25, 121–127. https://doi.org/10.12659/msmbr.914956

Upadhyay, J., S, N. N., Shetty, S., Saoji, A. A., & Yadav, S. S. (2023). Effects of Nadi Shodhana and Bhramari Pranayama on heart rate variability, auditory reaction time, and blood pressure: A randomized clinical trial in hypertensive patients. Journal of Ayurveda and Integrative Medicine, 14(4), 100774. https://doi.org/10.1016/j.jaim.2023.100774